Keto Mediterranean

A Beginner's Step-by-Step Guide W.
Meal Plan

Copyright © 2019 Bruce Ackerberg

All rights reserved

No part of this book may be reproduced, or stored in a retrieval system, or transmitted in any form or by any means, electronic, mechanical, photocopying, recording, or otherwise, without express written permission of the publisher.

Printed in the United States of America

Disclaimer

By reading this disclaimer, you are accepting the terms of the disclaimer in full. If you disagree with this disclaimer, please do not read the guide.

All of the content within this guide is provided for informational and educational purposes only, and should not be accepted as independent medical or other professional advice. The author is not a doctor, physician, nurse, mental health provider, or registered nutritionist/dietician. Therefore, using and reading this guide does not establish any form of a physician-patient relationship.

Always consult with a physician or another qualified health provider with any issues or questions you might have regarding any sort of medical condition. Do not ever disregard any qualified professional medical advice or delay seeking that advice because of anything you have read in this guide. The information in this guide is not intended to be any sort of medical advice and should not be used in lieu of any medical advice by a licensed and qualified medical professional.

The information in this guide has been compiled from a variety of known sources. However, the author cannot attest to or guarantee the accuracy of each source and thus should not be held liable for any errors or omissions.

You acknowledge that the publisher of this guide will not be held liable for any loss or damage of any kind incurred as a result of this guide or the reliance on any information provided within this guide. You acknowledge and agree that you assume all risk and responsibility for any action you undertake in response to the information in this guide.

Using this guide does not guarantee any particular result (e.g., weight loss or a cure). By reading this guide, you acknowledge that there are no guarantees to any specific outcome or results you can expect.

All product names, diet plans, or names used in this guide are for identification purposes only and are the property of their respective owners. The use of these names does not imply endorsement. All other trademarks cited herein are the property of their respective owners.

Where applicable, this guide is not intended to be a substitute for the original work of this diet plan and is, at most, a supplement to the original work for this diet plan and never a direct substitute. This guide is a personal expression of the facts of that diet plan.

Where applicable, persons shown in the cover images are stock photography models and the publisher has obtained the rights to use the images through license agreements with third-party stock image companies.

Table of Contents

Disclaimer	**2**
Introduction	**6**
Keto versus Mediterranean	**8**
The Keto Mediterranean Diet	**11**
Week 1 Learning Curve Week	**14**
Week 2 Preparation	**18**
Week 3 Making Your Meal Plan	**22**
Week 4 The Ketogenic Mediterranean Lifestyle	**25**
Selected Recipes	**28**
Smoked Salmon and Baked Eggs in Avocado	28
Keto Zucchini Walnut Bread	30
Egg Salad with Avocados	32
Tangy Lemon Fish	33
Spinach and Watercress Salad	35
Baked Salmon with Asparagus	36
Lemon Roasted Broccoli	37
Keto Zucchini Walnut Bread	38
Stuffed Chicken	40
Baked Salmon	41
Asian-Themed Macrobiotic Bowl	42
Avocado, Cucumber, and Tomato Salad	43
Tuna and Veggies Wrap	44
Chicken Salad	46
Keto Pesto Chicken	47
Conclusion	**49**
References and Helpful Links	**50**

Introduction

I want to thank you and congratulate you for getting this guide.

I know your first instinct is to ignore this guide and I can't blame you. I'm sure this is not the first guide you have seen about Diet and Nutrition nor am I the first to claim to have the best diet program. However, this guide is not just about diet and nutrition. This guide is more than just the best diet program. This is not just another guide about Keto diet and Mediterranean diet.

In my guide you will learn not just about diet and nutrition. With this guide, I will take you beyond learning about the best diet program. I will do more than give you information on Keto and Mediterranean diets. What I will do is walk with you on your journey as you start your way into becoming a healthier version of you.

We will discuss what Keto Mediterranean diet is all about, what benefits you will gain in using the diet and what food you should eat under this diet. Then we will walk together step-by-step how you can get started in this diet. I will not just give you a program. I will be there with you from start to finish. You will not be alone in this journey and along the way, I will share with you some tips, techniques and recipes to start you off.

You can't get any better deal than that. So, let's begin the journey together.

Thanks again for getting this guide. I hope you enjoy it!

Keto versus Mediterranean

Brief Overview of Mediterranean Diet
Mediterranean Diet is a diet based on the eating habits of people from Italy, Greece during the 1960's. The main characteristic of this diet is high consumption of olive oil, fruits, legumes, unrefined cereals and vegetables in proportions, a moderate to high consumption of fish and seafood, moderate consumption of dairy particularly cheese and yogurt, and wine; and low consumption of eggs and meat.

You could say that the Mediterranean Diet is more of an eating habit than a diet because there is no one single diet that you can follow because there are many countries around the Mediterranean continent and each may have eaten different foods.

Intensive research was done on the diet for more than 50 years but it was not until the Seven Countries Study by Professor Ancel Keys that the popularity of the Mediterranean diet soared. The macronutrient proportion of the Mediterranean diet used in the study consists 50% to 60% carbohydrates, 25% to 35% fats and the remainder is protein.

Common staple foods of the Mediterranean diet include vegetables, fruits, nuts, legumes, seeds, bread, potatoes, whole grains, fish, seafood, herbs and spices, and olive oil.

Brief Overview of the Keto Diet

The Keto diet is a very low carb, high fat, moderate to low protein diet. It was initially intended as treatment for cases of epilepsy in the early 1900s. The concept of the diet is to restrict carbs to the point that your body will enter the metabolic state of ketosis.

Metabolic state of Ketosis means your body is using ketones as alternative fuel or energy. The macronutrient proportion of the Keto diet is 70% fats, 25% protein and 5% carbohydrates.

Common staple foods of the Keto diet include meat, fish, poultry eggs, low carb vegetables, high fat dairy, nuts, seeds, avocado, berries, sweeteners, and other healthy fats.

Differences and Similarities
The keto and Mediterranean diets have different approaches but it is noteworthy to know their similarities and differences.

There are four major significant similarities between the two:
- Both diets give benefits to similar health areas like cholesterol levels, triglycerides levels, blood sugar levels, and blood pressure levels.
- Both diets focus on clean and healthy eating as both limit the consumption of processed food and derive most calories from whole foods.

- Both diets can provide almost the same weight loss result after one to two years.
- Both diets have the same dropout rates during dietary trials.

Despite its similarities, it is not without its differences:
- Ketogenic diets are very low carb including high carb plant foods while the Mediterranean diet includes moderately high carb foods despite its emphasis on healthy fats.
- When it comes to fat intake, the Mediterranean diet may be higher in fat intake compared with other diets but very low compared to Keto. Primary source of calorie for Keto is more of healthy fat but Mediterranean has its main source from carbohydrates
- Mediterranean emphasizes unsaturated fats from fish and plant-based oils while Keto is from unsaturated fats and copious amounts of saturated fats.

These similarities and differences when combined can both help improve your health despite their vast difference in approaches.

The Keto Mediterranean Diet

It was in 2008 that researchers in Spain explored the idea of combining the ketogenic diet and Mediterranean diet.

The diet plan included unlimited calories, olive oil as the main source of fat, vegetables and salads as main source of carbohydrates, fish for protein and a moderate amount of daily wine. The result yielded the same as that of a standard keto diet but the significant impact was the reduction of the LDL cholesterol and increase in HDL cholesterol.

Pitting the two diets against each other let us breakdown the benefits and downside of each diet and what is their common takeaway combined.

Benefits and Downside Keto and Mediterranean Diet

A comparative benefits and downside of each diet includes:

	Keto	Mediterranean
Benefits	✓ Increase in HDL cholesterol ✓ Reduce appetite and calorie consumption ✓ Eliminates food binge ✓ Reduce blood sugar, triglyceride, insulin levels ✓ Aids in treating Alzheimer's, Parkinson's, epilepsy, and type 2 diabetes'	✓ Health benefits is backed by more research ✓ Lowers risk of minerals and vitamins deficiency ✓ Significant decrease in LDL cholesterol ✓ Reduce cardiovascular disease ✓ Uses more environmentally friendly food
Downsides	✓ Has greater risk of mineral and vitamins deficiency ✓ Danger of keto flu ✓ Higher risk of unhealthy cholesterol levels ✓ Not good for people with thyroid condition	✓ Uses a wide variety of food that are prone to overeating ✓ Ineffective in key biomarkers for overall health

However, the one similar advantage of both diets when combined together is that it provides a significant increase in improving overall body composition and health compared with any other diet.

What is the Keto Mediterranean Diet

There is no specific definition for Keto Mediterranean diet but researches have shown that both diets and their macronutrient components have similar characteristics to promote health.

• Get most of the carbs from Keto friendly vegetables. Eat more leafy greens, cruciferous vegetables, and colorful vegetables. These vegetables contain fiber, minerals and vitamins that help optimize health and prevent symptoms of Keto flu

• Fish, poultry, seafood and eggs as primary sources of protein. These foods are rich not just with protein but unsaturated fats including omega 3.

• Restrict carbohydrates to promote ketosis. To enter ketosis, restrict carbs below 35 grams or below 25 grams of net carbs. This helps reduce your appetite and lower your levels of insulin, blood sugar, triglyceride and hbA1c.

• Consume plenty of polyunsaturated and monounsaturated fats. You can get these from olive oil, avocado oil, avocado, fish, seafood, nuts, dairy and seeds.

• Consume enough protein and fat depending on your goal. Your protein consumption if you are a bodybuilder is different from protein consumption of a normal person.

In essence, the Keto Mediterranean diet combines common Mediterranean foods with standard keto macronutrient targets to provide the body with the combined benefits of carb restriction, ketosis, whole foods and natural unsaturated fats.

Keto Mediterranean Food List

So what foods can you eat with a Keto Mediterranean diet?

Primary foods include:
- Mediterranean protein sources like fish, seafood, poultry, and eggs
- Fats and oil include avocado oil, olive oil and MCT oil
- Low carb fruits like olives, avocados, and tomatoes
- Low carb veggies like cruciferous vegetables, leafy greens and other low carb colorful vegetables
- Mediterranean flavorings like cumin, cinnamon oregano, paprika, anise, coriander, Spanish saffron, lemon and lime, mint garlic and others.

Moderate consumption:
- High fat dairy like full-fat cheese, yogurt, heavy cream
- Nuts and seeds like macadamia, pecans, brazil nuts, flax and chia
- Low carb fruits that includes melon and berries
- Saturated fats like coconut oil, ghee, butter and animal fats
- Red meat including beef, veal, lamb, pork

Food to Avoid
- Grains like wheat, rice, cereal, corn, etc.
- Legumes like black beans, lentils, peas, etc.
- Fruits like apples, oranges, bananas, etc.
- Tubers like potatoes, yams, etc.
- Sugar, which includes honey, maple, agave, etc.

Week 1 Learning Curve Week

With all that said, you are now good to go and start the combined Keto Mediterranean diet to a healthy new you.

If you are already on Keto diet, transitioning will just require a small amount of tweaking,

Step 1: Read, read, and read

This is the first step you need to do. This first step should be easy for you because in Chapters 1 and 2, I have already given you an overview of each diet and a comparative overview between the two.

Read all you can find about the diet. If you are new to the Ketogenic Diet, read all you can find about it. What makes it work, how you can succeed, what benefits the diet can give you. What kind of foods you can eat in Keto. If you are new to the diet, you can find information about the diet in books and in blog articles on the internet.

Then read on the Mediterranean diet. Get information about its history, its study, research breakthroughs made and what kind of foods you can eat under Mediterranean diet, then compare the two diets. Information is your basic tool so use it to your advantage.

Step 2: Assess your health condition?

Once you have all the information, make a personal assessment. Take stock of yourself. Find out the answers to the following questions:

- What is the current state of your health?
- Are you currently suffering from an illness?
- What kinds of illness are you suffering from?
- Is your blood pressure and sugar levels high?

Step 3: *Your physical stats*
Make a record of your physical stats.
- Record your weight and get your BMI. Is your BMI proportioned to your height and weight?
- What is your current cholesterol count?
- Record your blood sugar level. Is it normal or are you borderline diabetic?
- Is your blood pressure normal?

Step 4: *Do a healthy lifestyle check*
After assessing your health and your body, conduct if you are living a healthy lifestyle. Find out what is causing your problem. How bad or how good is your lifestyle? Are you living a healthy lifestyle?
- List down the foods that you regularly eat and your daily calorie intake.
- On your list of food, make a proportion of the macronutrients in your food. How much does the proportion of carbohydrates, fats, and protein contribute to your daily calorie intake?
- How much alcohol are you drinking? Are you drinking too much?
- Are you eating the right foods and getting the right macronutrients?
- Are you smoking?
- List your bad health habits to see what needs changing.

Step 5: Your paradigm shift

Once you are done, it is time to decide. You find that you are overweight, you have high blood sugar and cholesterol levels, and you are suffering from high blood pressure.

It's time to decide. What do you want to do? Do you want to lose weight? Do you want to lower your blood sugar level? Do you want to do both? Use this last step to decide which way you want to go. What is your next step?

Week 2 Preparation

Let's move to the second week, preparing yourself. You might want to ask why you need to prepare yourself. You cannot just start something without preparation. It would be like walking blindly into something and setting yourself up for failure.

Step 1: Setting your goal

Once you are ready to take the next step, plan your goal. Set your main goal and set small goals that would lead you to your main goals. Often, failure stems from the setting of goals. Identify what is your main goal, and then make realistic and achievable daily goals.

Be specific with your goal. If your goal is to lose weight, identify how much weight you want to lose. So, your main goal might look something like this:

"I want to lose 20 kilos in six months."

Once your main goal is set, start making smaller goals that would lead you to accomplish your main goal. You can make your small goals like this:
- Reduce my sweet intake.
- Eat ice cream once a week instead of everyday
- Shift to green and leafy vegetables instead of pasta

The above goals look realistic and achievable. Will it lead you to your ultimate goal? Yes. Will it be fast? Maybe yes, maybe no but it is realistic enough for you to know that you can achieve your goal without giving up.

Step 2: Cleaning your cupboard

Once you've listed down your goal, you can proceed to the next step. Cleaning up your cupboard. If you are not under any diet, chances are your food stock would consist of food you love to eat and these foods are usually high carb foods.

Do an inventory of your stock. If you have canned food, it would be best to donate it. The Keto Mediterranean diet is biased on whole foods and limits consumption of processed foods. Take out everything that is not acceptable under the diet.

If you are partial to a particular food, best find an alternative ingredient that would suit the diet. Junk the "cheat day" myth. You can eat even your favorite food without cheating on your diet.

Compare your inventory with the approved Keto Mediterranean food list. If it's not in there, then get rid of it.

Step 3: Making your food list

After your food inventory, make a list of the food you will need. List down ingredients that are friendly to your diet. List down foods that are Keto Mediterranean friendly. Since the diet is biased towards whole foods, you might already be buying some of them like fruits, meat, fish, dairy, vegetables, etc.

If you want food like bread or cereal, you might need to buy alternative ingredients to make them. To make bread, you can use almond flour or coconut flour instead of grain. Seeds and nuts are also good alternatives to oats or cereals.

Step 4: Working on your budget
You might need to replace your existing stock with a new diet but there are ways you can buy them without going broke. On your list, check which ones you can buy in bulk. Look for promo items or discounted items. Some ingredients cost less when bought in bulk.

Example, almond flour has many uses. You can make bread, pasta, cereals, etc. Buying it in bulk would be cheaper than buying it on a per need basis. Some foods you can stock for long periods in the fridge. Your vegetables you can buy fresh from farmers or wholesalers.

Step 5: Doing your purchases
For your initial purchase, it would be best to make your purchases moderate. Buy what you think you can consume in a week. You will make many adjustments on your diet as you go along and buying too much is not practical. You can stock up on ingredients once you have a fixed meal plan that works well for you.

Check the expiry dates of your purchases as well. If you are already buying in bulk, it is best to check for expiry dates so as not to waste a huge volume of ingredients in case it expires. You should also check your purchase quantities. If you are substituting ingredients, make sure you know the substitute ratio. This applies to any powder or liquid ingredients.

Week 3 Making Your Meal Plan

Time to make your meal plan.
Your meal plan is the list of food recipes you plan to eat for a specific length of time. The most popular are 7-days meal plan, 15-days meal plan and 30-days meal plan.

Step 1: Preparing your Meal plan
In this walk through, I have prepared a 5-day meal plan. We have incorporated our sample recipes in Chapter 7 in our meal plan.

Day 1
Breakfast: 1-2 serving of Flatbread
Lunch: 1-2 serving of Salmon lettuce with basil spread
Dinner: 1 serving of Tangy Lemon Fish
Side Dish: 1 serving of Lemon Roasted Broccoli

Day 2
Breakfast: 1-2 servings of Keto Cereal
Lunch: 2 servings of Egg salad with avocado
Dinner: 1 serving of stuffed chicken
Side Dish: 1 serving Slaw in avocado lime dressing

Day 3
Breakfast: 1-2 servings of Keto Zucchini Walnut Bread
Lunch: 1-2 servings Spinach watercress salad
Dinner: 1 serving of baked salmon
Side Dish: Pecan raspberry salad

Day 4

Breakfast: 1-2 servings of Baked eggs and cheese hash
Lunch: 1-2 serving of Egg salad with avocado
Dinner: 1 serving crusted salmon
Side Dish: 1 serving of Roasted Celery with Macadamia cheese

Day 5
Breakfast: 1-2 servings of Salmon breakfast bombs with hollandaise
Lunch: 1-2 servings of zucchini, avocado-walnut pesto salad
Dinner: 1 servings of shrimp salad
Side Dish: 1 serving of lemon roasted broccoli

This menu plan is merely a sample of a Keto Mediterranean diet. You can add dessert or other recipes depending on your preference. You can adapt Keto recipes and just add Mediterranean biased foods like olive oil, bitter vegetables, fish and dairy.

Step 2: Using what you currently have
When making your meal plan, check your inventory. See what ingredients you have and from there work on your meal plan. It is not advisable to prepare your meal plan then buy your stock afterwards.

The reason is if you cannot find the ingredient or if the ingredient is expensive, you will be forced to change your menu. You might end up spending more or wasting time changing your meal plan.

Step 3: Making Contingency Plans

You will not be eating at home all the time. There will be instances when you have to eat outside. Prepare a contingency plan so when it happens, you will not be caught red handed.

Keep a list of restaurants that are Keto friendly and suggest this to your friends and colleagues. If you are going on a business lunch or dinner and you are making the reservations, choose a Keto friendly restaurant. If you cannot do this, try to order food that is keto friendly.

When you are traveling, you can search for restaurants that cater to your diet. You can also take your own homemade snacks. Make advance arrangements with the hotel or place where you are staying.

Step 4: Making records of everything

Before you do your diet, record your body measurements and weight. If you are monitoring sugar levels and cholesterol levels, have a lab test to get the results and do another lab test after a week to measure changes.

A before and after record will help gauge if the diet is working for you or not.

Step 5: Rewarding yourself

Every success needs to be rewarded. Do not be stingy with yourself. Success is still success no matter how small it is. Rewarding yourself can help keep you motivated.

The reward does not have to be expensive. You can reward yourself with an extra serving of salad or allow yourself to have dessert as long as it remains within your dietary plan.

Week 4 The Ketogenic Mediterranean Lifestyle

You are on your fourth week. By this time, you have probably started or already midway to your new diet. By the end of the fourth week, you will be measuring the results of the diet.

Keep in mind the 7 pillars of the Keto Mediterranean diet to successfully achieve your goal and maintain a clean and healthy lifestyle.

1. Maintain low carb in your diet. Eat food that is low carb just like the Keto diet and combine with the Mediterranean low carb vegetables like bitter fruit and other cruciferous vegetables.

2. Prioritize green, leafy and colorful veggies. These fibrous veggies provide a plethora of healthy components to aid in stimulating the immune system. They contain fiber carbs that are acceptable in ketosis.

3. Eating more fat. Keto is a high fat diet but it has to be healthy fat and combining this with monounsaturated fat like olive oil, which is the focus of the Mediterranean diet.

4. Substitute sweet foods with cruciferous foods. These tend to help increase the defense system as compared with sweet foods. Sugar is glucose and glucose are carbohydrates. If you remove sugar, it will drastically lower down your glucose and insulin.

5. Exercise, exercise, exercise. Move your body. Even the best diets will only work best if you couple it with exercise. You don't need expensive equipment. Just increasing your physical activity is enough to help you exercise.

6. Aim for a long stretch between meals. Avoid snacking. Increasing the period without eating helps lower blood glucose and insulin. Although some diabetics need to have snacks in between meals, it is preferable if you eat healthy low carb snacks.

7. Apply the three R: Rest, Relaxation and Recovery. Your body can only take so much. Give it time to rest, relax and recover from stress and physical ravages. Apply the three R physically, mentally and spiritually.

Selected Recipes

In this Chapter, I'm sharing with you some of the Keto Mediterranean recipes that you can try out. These recipes are part of the sample Menu plan that we prepared in your walkthrough guide in Chapter 5.

Smoked Salmon and Baked Eggs in Avocado

Ingredients:
- 4 oz. smoked salmon
- 8 eggs
- 4 avocados, halved and deseeded
- fresh dill
- red chili flakes
- salt
- black pepper

Instructions:
1. Preheat the oven to 425°F.
2. In preparing the avocado, make sure that the hole where the seed was can fit an egg. Carve it out more if needed.
3. Place the avocados on a baking sheet.
4. Put smoked salmon strips on each hollow.
5. Crack open an egg in a small bowl. Spoon out the yolk and the white and transfer to the avocado. Carefully eyeball how much egg the avocado can hold.
6. Sprinkle the avocado with salt and pepper.
7. Bake in the oven for about 15-20 minutes.
8. Top with dill and chili flakes upon serving.

Keto Zucchini Walnut Bread

Ingredients:
- 3 large eggs
- 1/2 cup virgin olive oil
- 1 tsp. vanilla extract
- 2-1/4 cups fine almond flour
- 1-1/2 cups sweetener, erythritol
- 1/2 tsp. salt
- 1-1/2 tsp. baking powder
- 1/2 tsp. nutmeg, ground
- 1 tsp. cinnamon, ground
- 1/4 tsp. ginger, ground
- 1 cup zucchini, grated
- 1/2 cup walnuts, chopped

Instructions:
1. Preheat your oven to 350°F.
2. Whisk together the eggs, oil, and vanilla extract. Set aside.
3. Using another bowl, combine the baking powder, sweetener, almond flour, salt, cinnamon, nutmeg, and ginger powder. Set aside.
4. Squeeze the excess water from the zucchini using a paper towel or a cheesecloth.
5. Pour the zucchini into the egg mixture and whisk.
6. Add the flour mixture slowly into the egg and zucchini mixture. Blend using an electric blender until the mixture turns smooth.
7. Spray a loaf pan with avocado oil or baking spray.

8. Pour the zucchini batter into the loaf pan and smoothen the top evenly.

9. Spoon the chopped walnuts on top of the batter, lightly pressing the walnuts with the back of a spoon to press into the batter.

10. Pop the loaf pan into the oven and then bake for 60-70 minutes, or until the walnuts turn brown.

11. Cool in a cooling rack before slicing and serving.

Egg Salad with Avocados

Ingredients:
- 3 medium-sized avocados
- 6 eggs, large and hard-boiled
- 1/3 red onion, medium size
- 3 celery ribs
- 4 tbsp. mayonnaise
- 2 tbsp. freshly squeezed lime juice
- 2 tsp. brown mustard
- 1/2 tsp. cumin powder
- 1 tsp. hot sauce
- salt
- pepper

Instructions:
1. Chop the eggs, celery, and onion.
2. Set aside the avocados, then combine the rest of the ingredients.
3. Slice the avocado in half to take out the pit.
4. Stuff the avocado by spooning the egg salad on its cave.
5. Serve and enjoy.

Tangy Lemon Fish

Ingredients:
- 200 g. Gurnard fresh fish fillets
- 3 tbsp. butter
- 1 tbsp. fresh lemon juice
- 1/4 cup fine almond flour
- 1 tsp. dried dill
- 1 tsp. dried chives
- 1 tsp. onion powder
- 1/2 tsp. garlic powder
- salt
- pepper

Instructions:
1. On a large plate or tray, combine dill, almond flour, and spices. Mix until well combined.
2. Dredge each fillet one at a time into the flour mix. Turn the fillet around until fully coated, and then transfer to a clean plate or tray. This may be refrigerated until ready to cook.
3. Place a large pan over medium-high heat.
4. Combine halves of butter and lemon juice. Swirl the pan to mix, lift occasionally to avoid burning the butter.
5. Allow the fish to cook for about 3 minutes.
6. Let the fish absorb all the lemony-butter mixture. Cook on low heat to avoid drying out the pan.
7. Add the remaining lemon juice and butter to the pan.
8. Turn the fish to cook the other side for 3 minutes more. Swirl around the pan to fully coat it with the juice.

9. Wait until it turns golden brown and the fish is cooked through.
10. Serve with buttered vegetables.

Spinach and Watercress Salad

Ingredients:
- 1 cup watercress, washed with stems removed
- 3 cups baby spinach, washed with stems removed
- 1 medium sliced avocado
- 1/4 cup avocado oil
- 1/8 cup lemon juice
- a pinch of salt

Instructions:
1. Pat dry the spinach and watercress. Remove the stem and separate the leaves.
2. On a large serving plate, combine the leaves of the watercress and the spinach.
3. Cut the avocado in half, then remove the pit. Peel the skin off from each side.
4. Slice the avocados into thin strips. Set aside.
5. Prepare the dressing by combining avocado oil and lemon juice.
6. Arrange the avocado strips on top of the watercress and spinach.
7. Season with salt and pepper.
8. Drizzle with the dressing before serving.

Baked Salmon with Asparagus

Ingredients:
- 1.5 lbs. wild salmon
- 2 tbsp. olive oil
- 3 cloves garlic, minced
- 1 tsp. dried oregano
- pepper
- sea salt
- 1 bunch fresh asparagus
- 1/2 cup cucumber
- 1/2 cup tomato, diced
- 1/2 cup feta cheese
- 1/2 cup olives
- 1 whole lemon

Instructions:
1. Preheat the oven to 400°F.
2. Use parchment paper to line a baking sheet. Set aside.
3. Mix oil, oregano, salt, garlic, and pepper in a bowl.
4. Pour seasoning mix over the salmon and coat the entire fish.
5. Layer the salmon on the baking sheet.
6. Place trimmed asparagus on the sheet pan next to the salmon.
7. Squeeze fresh lemon juice and place the remaining lemon slices on the sheet pan. Bake for 20 minutes.
8. When the salmon is done, serve with a scoop of olive & feta salad over the salmon or on the side and serve.

Lemon Roasted Broccoli

Ingredients:
- 1-1/2 lb. broccoli florets
- 1/3 cup shredded Parmesan cheese
- 1/4 cup olive oil
- 2 tbsp. fresh basil, chopped
- 3 tsp. minced garlic
- 1/2 – 3/4 tsp. kosher salt
- 1/2 tsp. red chili flakes
- 1/2 lemon juice and zest

Instructions:
1. Preheat the oven to 425°F.
2. Line a baking sheet with parchment paper and spread the broccoli florets.
3. Season the broccoli with basil, olive oil, garlic, kosher salt, chili flakes, lemon zest, and lemon juice.
4. Sprinkle the top with parmesan cheese then put into the oven for 20-25 minutes or until the cheese has slightly melted.
5. Serve and enjoy while warm.

Keto Zucchini Walnut Bread

Ingredients:
- 3 large eggs
- 1/2 cup virgin olive oil
- 1 tsp. vanilla extract
- 2-1/4 cups fine almond flour
- 1-1/2 cups sweetener, erythritol
- 1/2 tsp. salt
- 1-1/2 tsp. baking powder
- 1/2 tsp. nutmeg, ground
- 1 tsp. cinnamon, ground
- 1/4 tsp. ginger, ground
- 1 cup zucchini, grated
- 1/2 cup walnuts, chopped

Instructions:
1. Preheat your oven to 350°F.
2. Whisk together the eggs, oil, and vanilla extract. Set aside.
3. Using another bowl, combine the baking powder, sweetener, almond flour, salt, cinnamon, nutmeg, and ginger powder. Set aside.
4. Squeeze the excess water from the zucchini using a paper towel or a cheesecloth.
5. Pour the zucchini into the egg mixture and whisk.
6. Add the flour mixture slowly into the egg and zucchini mixture. Blend using an electric blender until the mixture turns smooth.
7. Spray a loaf pan with avocado oil or baking spray.

8. Pour the zucchini batter into the loaf pan and smoothen the top evenly.
9. Spoon the chopped walnuts on top of the batter, lightly pressing the walnuts with the back of a spoon to press into the batter.
10. Pop the loaf pan into the oven and then bake for 60-70 minutes, or until the walnuts turn brown.
11. Cool in a cooling rack before slicing and serving.

Stuffed Chicken

Ingredients:
- 4 pcs. chicken breast filets, skinless and boneless
- 1/4 cup feta cheese, crumbled
- 1/4 cup artichoke hearts, finely chopped, drained, and marinated
- 2 tbsp. red peppers, finely chopped, drained, and roasted
- 2 tbsp. green onion, thinly sliced
- 2 tsp. fresh oregano, or 1/2 tsp. if using dried oregano
- 1 tsp. kosher salt
- 1/4 tsp. ground black pepper

Instructions:
1. Cut a pocket in each chicken breast using a sharp knife. Cut through the thickest portion horizontally without cutting through the opposite side.
2. Combine the feta, roasted peppers, artichoke hearts, oregano and green onions into a mixture.
3. Fill each pocket of the chicken breast with the mixture.
4. Close the opening of the pockets with a wooden toothpick.
5. Season the chicken breast with salt and pepper.
6. Preheat a non-stick large skillet on medium heat.
7. Coat it with cooking spray.
8. Fry the chicken for 10 to 12 minutes on each side, or until the internal temperature reaches at least 165°F.
9. Serve hot.

Baked Salmon

Ingredients:
- 2 salmon fillets
- 6 cups of fresh spinach
- 2 tsp. coconut oil
- 1/4 tsp. garlic powder
- 1/4 tsp. turmeric
- 3 large cloves of garlic
- lemon juice
- salt
- pepper

Instructions:
1. Preheat the oven to 400°F.
2. Line a baking dish with parchment paper.
3. Marinate salmon fillets in lemon juice, coconut oil, garlic powder, turmeric, salt, and pepper.
4. Let it sit for a few minutes. This may also be done the night before to help the juices and flavor get into the salmon.
5. Once the oven is ready, bake the salmon for 15 minutes.
6. Cook some of the garlic in a pan with coconut oil.
7. Add spinach and cook until ready. Season with salt and pepper to taste.
8. Take salmon out of the oven and put spinach beside it.
9. Serve and enjoy.

Asian-Themed Macrobiotic Bowl

Ingredients:
- 2 cups cooked quinoa
- 4 carrots
- 1 package of smoked tofu
- 1 tbsp. nutritional yeast
- 2 tbsp. coconut aminos
- 4 tbsp. sunflower sprouts
- 2 tbsp. fermented vegetables
- 1 cup of shiitake mushrooms
- 1 avocado
- 2 tbsp. hemp seeds
- 2-3 cooked beets
- coconut oil cooking spray

Dressing:
- 2 tbsp. miso paste
- 1 tbsp. tahini
- 1 clove of garlic, crushed
- 1 tbsp. olive oil
- 1/2 lime, juiced
- 3 tbsp. water

Instructions:
1. Roast the carrots in the oven at 400°F for 30-40 minutes.
2. Wash the vegetables, trim, and spray them with coconut oil.
3. Add them to the oven. When they are cooked, set them aside till you are ready to assemble the Buddha bowl.

4. Make the dressing by combining all of the ingredients in a medium-sized bowl. If the dressing appears lumpy, add more water.
5. To build the bowl, put the quinoa on the bottom and then arrange the vegetables on top.
6. Sprinkle the bowls with hemp seeds and drizzle the dressing over top upon serving.

Avocado, Cucumber, and Tomato Salad

Ingredients:
- 1/4 cup extra-virgin olive oil
- 1 pc. lemon, juiced
- 1/4 tsp. cumin, ground
- salt, to taste
- freshly ground black pepper, to taste
- 3 medium avocados, cubed
- 1-pint cherry tomatoes, halved
- 1 small cucumber, sliced into half-moons
- 1/3 cup corn
- 2 tbsp. cilantro, chopped

Instructions:
1. Combine avocados, cilantro, corn, cucumber, jalapeño, and tomatoes in a large bowl.
2. In a separate small container, whisk together lemon juice, cumin, and oil to make the salad dressing.
3. Season the dressing with salt and pepper.
4. Toss the salad gently while adding the dressing.
5. Serve immediately.

Tuna and Veggies Wrap

Ingredients:
- 1 canned tuna
- 2 pcs. whole-grain tortillas
- 1 cup cucumber, sliced
- 1 tbsp. low-fat Italian dressing
- 1 cup carrots, julienned

Instructions:
1. Put the dressing and tuna in a bowl and mix well.
2. Arrange half of the mixture on one of the tortillas. Add half the amount of each vegetable and wrap.
3. Do the same to the remaining tortilla.

Chicken Salad

Ingredients:
- 1 small can of premium chunk chicken breast packed in water
- 1 stalk celery, large, finely chopped
- 1/4 cup reduced-fat mayonnaise
- 4 romaine leaves or red leaf lettuce, washed and trimmed
- 8 pcs. cherry tomatoes or 1 ripe tomato, quartered
- 1 cucumber, small and sliced thinly

Instructions:
1. Drain canned chicken and transfer to a bowl.
2. Put in celery and mayonnaise.
3. Mix lightly. Don't crush the chicken.
4. In a separate shallow bowl, place the lettuce neatly.
5. Add the chicken salad in the middle
6. Add tomatoes and cucumber slices to the plate.
7. Refrigerate before serving, cover with plastic wrap.

Keto Pesto Chicken

Ingredients:
- 1-1/2 lbs chicken thighs breasts, boneless and cut into bite-sized pieces
- pepper
- salt
- 2 tbsp. butter or coconut oil
- 5 tbsp. red or green pesto
- 1-1/4 cups heavy whipping cream
- 5 oz. feta cheese, diced
- 3 oz. pitted olives
- 1 garlic clove, finely chopped

Salad:
- 5 oz. leafy greens
- 4 tbsp. olive oil
- sea salt
- ground black pepper

Instructions:
1. Preheat the oven to 400°F.
2. Season the chicken with salt and pepper.
3. Add butter or oil to a large skillet. Fry the chicken pieces on medium-high heat until golden brown.
4. In a bowl, combine heavy cream and pesto. Mix well.
5. Put the fried chicken meat in a baking dish. Add in olives, garlic, and feta cheese.
6. Pour the pesto or cream mixture.
7. Bake in the oven for 20-30 minutes.
8. Toss all the salad ingredients upon serving.

9. Serve and enjoy.

Conclusion

Thank you again for getting this guide!

Now you have a clearer understanding of the Ketogenic Mediterranean diet. I hope that my walkthrough guide has helped you make the next step towards a cleaner and healthier lifestyle.

The guide is not set on stone. It is merely a starting point for you and as you move along, you can adjust it to suit your lifestyle. The important thing is you have taken the next step.

If you found this guide helpful, please take the time to share your thoughts and post a review. It would be greatly appreciated!

Thank you and good luck!

References and Helpful Links

30-day low-carb mediterranean diet meal plan. (n.d.). EatingWell. Retrieved May 20, 2023, from https://www.eatingwell.com/article/7869888/30-day-low-carb-mediterranean-diet-meal-plan/

Manager, C. (n.d.). What is the mediterranean keto diet? Carb Manager. Retrieved May 20, 2023, from https://www.carbmanager.com/article/yel2oraaaiawrknu/what-is-the-mediterranean-keto-diet

nina.bai@stanford.edu, <img src='https://med stanford edu/news/media-contacts/nina-bai/_jcr_content/image img 620 high jpg/Nina-Bai2 jpg' alt='Nina Bai'> Nina Bai Nina Bai is a science writer in the Office of Communications Email her at. (2022, June 15). Keto and Mediterranean diets both help manage diabetes, but one is easier to maintain. News Center. http://med.stanford.edu/news/all-news/2022/070/keto-mediterranean-diet-diabetes.html

Pérez-Guisado, J., Muñoz-Serrano, A., & Alonso-Moraga, Á. (2008). Spanish Ketogenic Mediterranean diet: A healthy cardiovascular diet for weight loss. Nutrition Journal, 7(1), 30. https://doi.org/10.1186/1475-2891-7-30

The mediterranean keto diet: Food list, sample meal plan, and recipes - perfect keto. (n.d.). Retrieved May 20,

2023, from https://perfectketo.com/mediterranean-keto-diet/

Printed in Great Britain
by Amazon